Mediterranean Sweet Wonders

A Sweet Collection of Unmissable Desserts from the Mediterranean

Valerie Reynolds

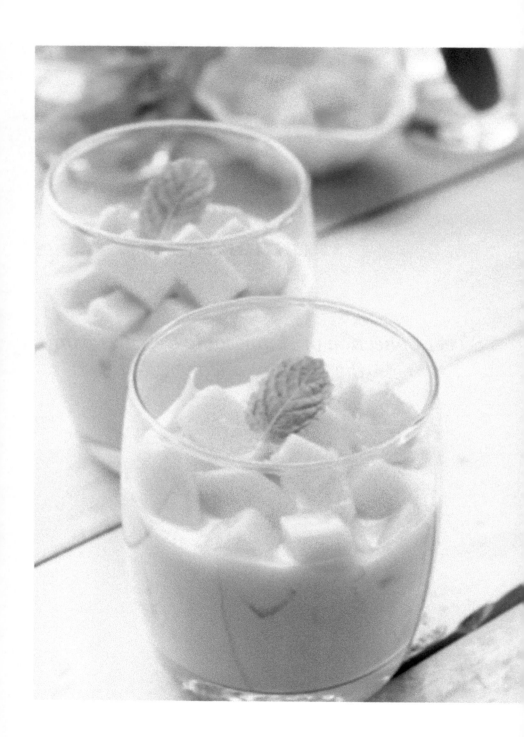

By reading this document, the reader agrees that under no circumstances is the author responsible for any losses, direct or indirect, which are incurred as a result of the use of information contained within this document, including, but not limited to, — errors, omissions, or inaccuracies.

Table of Contents

6

Lemon lime cucumber water

It is a perfect alternative to quenching you thirst to taking water. It is entirely sugar free making vegetarian. This recipe also helps to chop weight and detox the body.

Ingredients

- 4 cups Water
- 2 Limes
- 12 slices Lemon
- 16 slices Cucumber

Directions

- Combine sliced lemon, lime, and cucumber in a jar.
- Pour water over the jar and cover tightly.
- Allow the water to infuse in a refrigerator for 4 hours.
- Serve and enjoy.

Muddled mint and cucumber cooler cocktail

Ingredients

- 1 small cucumber, sliced
- 1 oz. gin
- ¼ cup of fresh mint leaves
- 1 cup of lemonade
- Ice

Directions

- Begin by muddling 4 slices of cucumber with the mint in a shaker together with the ice, lemonade and gin.
- Shake well and pour into a tall 8-ounce glass.
- Garnish with extra cucumber slices and mint leaves.
- Serve and enjoy.

Mint lemonade

Mint lemonade gives a refreshing taste to this recipe blended with lemon juice. In 5 minutes your juice will be ready.

Ingredients

- 6 mint sprigs
- 4 cups of water
- 3 lemons
- 3 tablespoons of granulated sugar

Directions

- Pour water in a large pitcher.
- Add sugar and freshly squeezed juice from 2 lemons.
- Stir to dissolved the sugar.
- Then, add the mint sprigs together with the lemon slices.
- Cover the pitcher with the lid.
- Refrigerate for 2 hours.
- Serve and enjoy.

Pineapple infused water

This is a method of replenishing the lost water in your body especially if you do not prefer to take water. But it is recommended to take natural water anyway.

Ingredients

- 2 – 4 Sprigs Mint
- 1 Pineapple
- 4 cups Water

Directions

- Cut the pineapple and slice thinly.
- Dice the juicy flesh.
- Place in a jug.
- Add a bit of mint sprigs with water.
- Cover well and refrigerate to let infuse overnight.
- Strain the water and keep refrigerated.
- Serve and enjoy.

Spinach cucumber smoothie

If you lack vitamins and antioxidants in your diet, make sure your boost them with this recipe because they are rich in these food values.

Ingredients

- 8 <u>pitted dates</u>
- 1 cucumber
- 1 medium apple
- 1 avocado
- 1½ cup of spinach, packed
- 2 cups almond milk

Directions

- Peel and dice both the apple and the cucumber.
- Cut the avocado in half, remove the seed.
- Chop the dates roughly.
- Combine all the ingredients in a blender.
- Let blend until smooth.

Watermelon beet juice

Watermelon with beet is a perfect Mediterranean Sea diet fruit combination for total hydration and boosting of blood supply by the beet. It is quite refreshing.

Ingredients

- Mint
- 2 Medium Beets
- 2.5 pounds Watermelon
- Lemon

Directions

- Prepare the fruits by washing and peeling.
- Place all of them in a blender.
- Blends until every flesh is crushed into juice.
- Taste and adjust accordingly with the lemon.
- Garnish with mint and watermelon wedge, if you like.
- Serve and enjoy immediately.
- Refrigerate the balance.

Immune boosting turmeric tea

Take charge of your immunity health by making this Mediterranean magical recipe. It blends in turmeric root, mind and ginger flavors.

Ingredients

- A pinch of black pepper , per cup
- 2 cups water
- 2 – 3 fresh mint sprigs
- 1 thumb size ginger root
- 1 orange, small
- 1 thumb size turmeric root

Directions

- Firstly, start by boiling water.
- Clean the turmeric, ginger, orange, and mint; peel and slice the turmeric and ginger. Cut the orange into half.
- Divide ingredients in 2 mugs.
- Add in boiling water over it.
- Add a pinch of black pepper.
- Squeeze orange juice (a little bit).
- Allow it to steep for 15 minutes.

- Serve and drink.

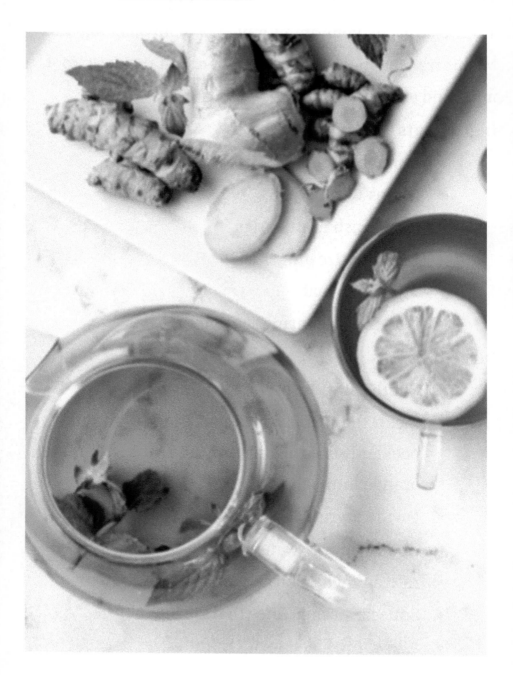

Watermelon juice with grapes

This recipe combines mint with honey, grapes and some extra flavor.

Ingredients

- 10 white grapes
- 4 cups of watermelon pieces
- Ice cubes
- 2 tablespoons of freshly squeezed lemon juice
- 3 tablespoons of honey
- 10 mint leaves

Directions

- Cut watermelon into chunks.
- Place in a blender along with the mint leaves and blend to combine.
- Place into glasses together with grapes, ice cubes and garnish with mint.
- Serve and enjoy immediately.

Orange infused water

With turmeric and citrus flavor this Mediterranean Sea diet recipe is a perfect choice to quench your thirst. It is tasty and very refreshing.

Ingredients

- 4 cups of water
- 4 basil sprigs
- 1 large orange
- 2 turmeric roots

Directions

- Wash and slice the orange.
- Peel and slice turmeric roots.
- Place water in a large jug.
- Add the orange slices together with the turmeric and basil.
- Cover and chill in the fridge for 12 hours.
- Serve and enjoy.

Energy boosting smoothie with papaya and avocado

This recipe is a bomb blast of vitamin, fiber with immunity boosting properties. The can get a sufficient energy from this Mediterranean fruity diet recipe.

Ingredients

- 2 Oranges
- 1 lb. Papaya
- 1 Banana
- 1 Avocado

Directions

- Peel all the fruits, remove seeds and chop into chinks.
- Place everything a food processor.
- Squeeze orange juice in it.
- Process until smooth.
- Serve in your glass and enjoy immediately.

Cloudy apple pear juice

Ingredients

- 6 Apples
- 3 Pears

Directions

- Cut apples and pears, after cleaning, into quarters and core them.
- Juice both in a juicer.
- Serve and enjoy.

712. Orange Julius

Oranges are used with milk and vanillas to make this healthy and tasty juice. You can use any sweetener to add more sweet taste if needed.

Ingredients

- 1 teaspoon of Vanilla Extract
- 1/4 cup Milk
- 6 Oranges, medium-large
- 2 tablespoons of Maple Syrup
- 1 cup Ice

Directions

- Squeeze the juice out of the oranges.

- Place in a blender.
- Add ice together with milk, maple syrup, and vanilla extract.
- Blend until smooth and creamy.
- Serve in glasses and enjoy immediately.

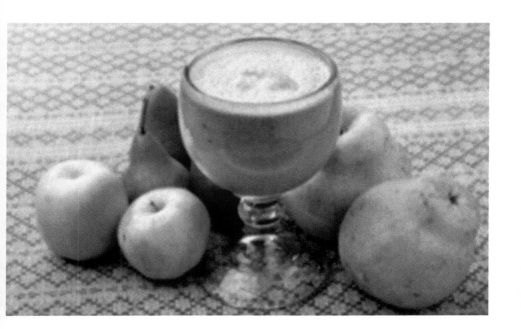

Watermelon Agua Fresca

This is a sugar free recipe with low calorie content. It is fresh and refreshing especially during summer times.

Ingredients

- 2 teaspoons of <u>maple syrup</u>
- 6 cups of watermelon chunks
- 5 teaspoons of fresh lemon juice
- 1 cup of water

Directions

- In a blender, put all the ingredients except lemon juice.
- Blend until ready.
- Add 5 teaspoons lemon juice, stir.
- Taste and adjust accordingly.
- Strain, serve and enjoy.

Basic blueberry smoothie

This basic blueberry smoothie is a very luscious breakfast recipe with high nutrition content. It is highly creamy made with frozen blueberries, almond milk and butter as well as bananas.

Ingredients

- 1/4 cup of almond butter
- 1 ½ cups of to 2 cups unsweetened vanilla almond milk or water
- 2 teaspoons of maple syrup, if necessary
- 1 ½ cups of frozen blueberries
- 1 ½ cup of frozen bananas

Directions

- In a blender, combine all of the ingredients.
- Blend gently and increase gradually.
- Continue blending up to the highest blender speed.
- Keep scarping the mixture from the sides of the blender.
- You can add more milk at this point if you like.

- After the smoothie is very creamy, feel free to taste.
- You can then add the maple syrup in case you prefer a sweeter smoothie.
- Divide the smoothie into glasses.
- Serve immediately and enjoy.

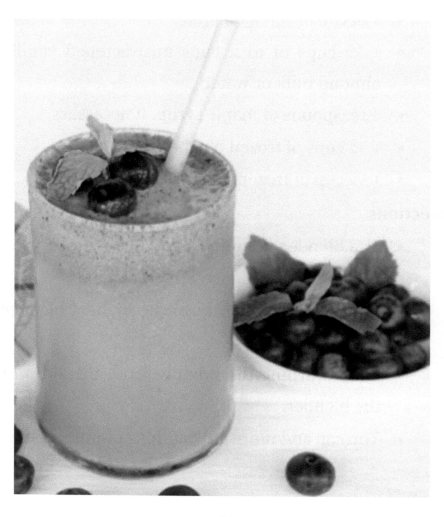

Banana almond smoothie

This Mediterranean Sea diet recipe per harps takes the shortest time to prepare. In 5 minutes or less, your creamy banana smooth will just be ready to quench your appetite for it.

Ingredients

- ½ cup of almond milk, yogurt
- 1 medium to large frozen banana
- Tiny drop of almond extract
- 1 heaping spoonful of almond butter
- Drizzle of honey, agave nectar
- 2 spoonfuls of flax seed

Directions

- Toss all the ingredients into a blender at once and blend until smooth or to your liking.
- Pour into a glass
- Enjoy.

Mediterranean Sea diet soup recipes

Roasted tomato basil soup

The roasted tomato recipe derived its delicacy power from aromatic fresh herbs especially thyme and other spices. The use of extra virgin olive oil propels it to the next level of a wonderful finish with a heavy cream.

Ingredients

- 2 to 3 carrots peeled and cut into small chunks
- 5 garlic cloves minced
- ½ teaspoon of ground cumin
- 2 ½ cups water
- 1 teaspoon of dry oregano
- Salt and pepper
- Extra virgin olive oil
- ½ teaspoon of paprika
- 2 medium yellow onions chopped
- 1 cup canned crushed tomatoes
- 2 oz. fresh basil leaves
- 3 lb. Roma tomatoes halved
- Splash of lime juice optional
- 3 – 4 fresh thyme springs 2 tsp thyme leaves

Directions

- Heat oven ready to 450°.
- Combine tomatoes and carrot pieces in a large mixing bowl.
- Drizzle the extra virgin olive oil over it, then season with kosher salt and black pepper.
- Toss to combine.
- Change to a large baking sheet and spread well in one layer.
- Roast in the heated oven for 30 minutes.
- Remove when ready from the heat and set keep aside for 10 minutes to allow cooling.
- Move the roasted tomatoes along with the carrots to a food processor fitted with a blade.
- Add little water for blending.
- Heat 2 tablespoon of extra virgin olive oil over medium-high temperature until it shimmers in a large cooking pot.
- Introduce the onions and cook for 3 minutes.
- Introduce the garlic and cook shortly until golden.

- Pour the roasted tomato mixture into the cooking pot.
- Stir in the crushed tomatoes, basil, spices, thyme and ½ of water
- Season with a little kosher salt and black pepper.
- Boil, then reduce the heat and cover part-way to let simmer for 20 minutes.
- Remove the thyme springs and transfer tomato basil soup to serving bowls.
- Serve with crusty bread and enjoy.

Quinoa vegetables soup

This is purely a Mediterranean Sea diet soup feature with several variety of vegetables, herbs and quinoa. Gluten free, it is a perfect healthy option for you.

Ingredients

- 2 celery stalks, chopped
- 6 garlic cloves, minced
- 1 large can of diced tomatoes
- 3 carrots, peeled and chopped
- 2 cups of chopped vegetables
- Scant 1 cup of quinoa, rinsed
- 4 cups of vegetable broth
- 2 cups of water
- 1 medium onion, chopped
- 1 teaspoon of salt
- 2 bay leaves
- Pinch red pepper flakes
- 3 tablespoons of extra virgin olive oil
- Ground black pepper
- 1 can of great northern beans
- 1 cup of chopped fresh kale

- 2 teaspoons of lemon juice
- ½ teaspoon of dried thyme

Directions

- Warm olive oil in a large oven over medium heat till shimmering.
- Add carrot, chopped onion, seasonal vegetables, celery, and a pinch of salt.
- Let cook as you stir frequently, until onion are translucent in 6 – 8 minutes.
- Add garlic together with thyme.
- Cook until fragrant while stirring frequently in 1 minute.
- Stir in the diced tomatoes cook for briefly minutes, stirring frequently.
- Pour in the broth, quinoa, and the water.
- Add 2 bay leaves, 1 teaspoon of salt, and a pinch of red pepper flakes.
- Season with ground black pepper.
- Increase the heat let boil.
- Partially cover the pot and reduce heat to let simmer for 25 minutes.
- Add beans along with chopped greens.

- Simmering for 5 minutes.
- Take off heat, remove the bay leaves.
- Stir in 1 teaspoon lemon juice.
- Taste and season accordingly.
- Divide into bowls.
- Serve and enjoy.

Mediterranean spicy spinach lentil soup

Ingredient

- 2 cups chopped flat leaf parsley
- Greek Extra Virgin Olive Oil
- 1 ½ teaspoon of sumac
- 6 cups low-sodium vegetable broth
- 1 large garlic clove, chopped
- Salt and pepper
- 1 ½ cups green lentils or small brown lentils
- Pinch of sugar
- 1 large yellow onion, chopped
- 1 ½ teaspoon of ground cumin
- 12 oz. frozen cut leaf spinach
- 1 ½ teaspoon of crushed red peppers
- 2 teaspoon of dried mint flakes
- 3 cups water, more if needed
- 1 ½ teaspoon of ground coriander
- 1 lime juice
- 1 tablespoon flour

Directions

- In a large <u>cast iron pot</u> , heat 2 tablespoon of olive oil.
- Add the chopped onions and continue to Sauté until turns golden brown.
- Introduce the garlic, dried mint, flour, sugar, and all the spices and cook for 2 minutes over medium heat, keep stirring frequently.
- Add broth and water.
- Increase the heat to high enough to bring the liquid to a rolling boil
- Introduce the frozen spinach and the lentils to the content.
- On a high temperature cook for 5 minutes.
- Lower the heat to medium cook for 20 minutes when covered.
- When the lentils are fully cooked, stir in the lime juice and chopped parsley.
- Remove from the heat cover and let settle for 5 minutes.
- Serve hot with pita bread.

Simple mushroom barley soup

Seeking for a deliciously comfortable vegetable soup? This simple mushroom soup is the perfect answer with perfect flavors and subtle smoky finish.

Ingredients

- Black pepper
- Extra virgin olive oil
- 2 celery stalks, chopped
- 1 yellow onion, chopped
- Kosher salt
- 1 cup pearl barley rinsed
- ½ - 3/4 teaspoon of smoked paprika
- 4 garlic cloves, chopped
- 8 ounces of white mushrooms, cleaned and chopped
- ½ cup canned crushed tomatoes
- 1 teaspoon of coriander
- ½ teaspoon of cumin
- 6 cups low-sodium broth
- 1 carrot, chopped
- ½ cup packed chopped parsley

- 16 ounces of baby Bella mushrooms, sliced

Directions

- In a large oven, heat extra virgin olive oil over medium-high temperature to shimmer without smoke.
- Add baby bell mushrooms and cook until mushrooms soften to gain some color in approximately 5 minutes thereabout.
- Remove from the pot and keep aside.
- Using the same pot, add small extra virgin olive oil.
- Add onions, celery, chopped white mushrooms, and carrots, then let cook for 4 – 5 minutes over medium temperature.
- Season with the salt and pepper.
- Introduce the crushed tomatoes and coriander, smoked paprika, and cumin.
- Let cook for 3 minutes, keep tossing frequently.
- Add both the broth and pearl barley.
- Bring to a rolling boil for 5 minutes

- Remove the heat let simmer over low temperature for 45 minutes until tender or cooked through.
- Transfer the cooked Bella mushrooms back to the pot and stir to blend.
- Continue to cook for 5 minutes to warm the mushrooms through.
- Finish with fresh parsley.
- Serving in bowls.
- Enjoy.

Cold cucumber soup

Ingredients

- Lemon juice
- Salt, to taste
- 2 pounds of fresh cucumbers, peeled and diced
- ¼ cup fresh parsley, chopped
- ½ cup fresh dill, chopped
- 1 cup Greek yogurt
- Black pepper
- ½ cup water
- 1 medium onion, quartered

Directions

- In a blender, combine diced cucumbers together with the Greek yogurt, pinch of black pepper, dill, onion, chopped parsley, salt and water. Blend until smooth.
- Taste and adjust accordingly.
- Drizzle some lemon juice over and blend again.
- Serve and enjoy chilled.

Red pepper and walnut dip

Ingredients

- 2 teaspoon of cumin powder
- 1 clove of garlic
- The juice of half a lemon
- 2/3 cup of chopped walnuts
- ¼ teaspoon of cayenne powder
- 1 cup of chopped roasted red bell peppers
- 4 tablespoons of tomato paste
- 2 tablespoons of extra virgin olive oil
- ¼ cup of rolled oats

Directions

- Place all the ingredients in a food processor.
- Blend until smooth.
- Serve and enjoy.

Simple Italian minestrone soup

The Italian minestrone soup is perfectly brimmed with variety of vegetables, pasta, and beans. The thick flavorful tomato broth with some rosemary and herbs gives this soup a total draw.

Ingredients

- 1 small yellow onion chopped
- 2 celery stalks diced
- Salt and pepper
- Large handful chopped parsley
- 2 carrots chopped
- 1pinch Parmesan cheese rind optional
- 1/4 cup of extra virgin olive oil
- 6 cups of broth vegetable or chicken broth
- 1 15 ounces can kidney beans
- 4 garlic cloves minced
- 1 cup green beans fresh
- ½ teaspoon of rosemary
- Grated Parmesan cheese to serve (optional)
- 1 15 ounces of can crushed tomatoes
- 1 teaspoon of paprika

- 2 – 3 springs fresh thyme
- Handful fresh basil leaves
- 1 zucchini or dices yellow squash
- 1 bay leaf
- 2 cups of cooked small pasta

Directions

- In a large oven, heat the extra virgin olive oil over medium heat until shimmering without smoke.
- Add carrots, onions, and celery.
- Increase the heat to medium-high let cook while tossing regularly until the veggies soften somehow for 5 minutes.
- Add the garlic continue to cook for more 5 minutes, keep tossing.
- Add the zucchini or yellow squash and green beans the content.
- Season with rosemary, paprika, and a generous pinch of kosher salt and pepper, then toss to combine.
- Add the broth, crushed tomatoes, bay leaf, fresh thyme, and Parmesan rind.

- Boil, then reduce the heat to let simmer for 20 minutes covering the pot partially.
- Uncover the pot to add the kidney beans let cook for 5 – 10 minutes.
- Stir in the parsley and fresh basil at once.
- Stir in the cooked pasta and simmer briefly till the pasta is warmed through, if you want to serve immediately. Ensure not to overcook.
- Remove the cheese rind and bay leaf.
- Taste and adjust seasoning accordingly to your taste.
- Serve the minestrone when hot in dinner bowls and then sprinkle with grated Parmesan which is optional.
- Enjoy

Tomato gazpacho soup

Tomato gazpacho soup blends variety of fresh vegetables with flavorful appetizers. Garlic and onion gives this recipe the desired taste and aroma.

Ingredients

- 1 cucumber
- 1/4 cup of water
- 2 tablespoon of extra virgin olive oil
- 1 small onion
- A pinch of black pepper
- 1 green pepper
- 2 small slices of sourdough bread
- 1 garlic clove
- 2 tablespoon of apple vinegar
- 2.2 pounds of ripe tomatoes
- 1/4 tablespoon of salt

Directions

- Boil water in a pot.
- Place tomatoes the boiling water till the skin starts coming off.
- Remove the tomatoes let them cool down.

- Peel off the softened tomato skin and dice.
- Combine and place vegetables and bread in the blender.
- Blend until all ingredients until smooth.
- Taste and adjust accordingly.
- Serve and enjoy with a drizzle of oil.

5-ingredients spring vegetable soup

This spring vegetable is readily available all year round. It is light, purely vegetarian for a perfect Mediterranean Sea diet with vitamin boosting properties.

Ingredients

- 1 vegetable stock cube
- 2 tablespoon of sunflower oil
- 2 large potatoes
- 3 medium carrots
- 1 cup of frozen
- 3 celery stalks
- 1 small onion
- Salt

Directions

- Dice your onion peeled.
- Sauté for 4 minutes while stirring infrequently over medium heat.
- Add sliced carrots, celery, potatoes as well as peas to a pot.
- Sauté for briefly, then add 1.5 liter of water.
- Season with salt.

- Bring to boil.
- Place in vegetable stock cube over reduced heat.
- Cook for 30 minutes.
- Serve and enjoy.

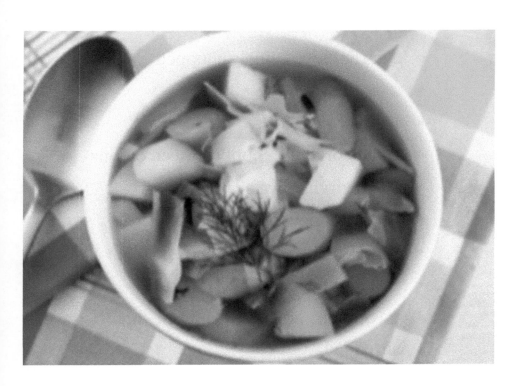

Greek avgolemono soup

This recipe is a lemon flavored egg made into a soup with broth and it is highly fragrant and silky.

Ingredients

- 2 large eggs
- ½ cup of finely chopped carrots
- ½ cup of finely chopped celery
- 2 garlic cloves, finely chopped
- 2 bay leaves
- 1 cup of rice
- ½ cup of finely chopped green onions
- Extra virgin olive oil
- Fresh parsley for garnish
- 8 cups of low-sodium chicken broth
- Salt and pepper
- 2 cooked boneless chicken breast pieces, shredded
- ½ cup of freshly-squeezed lemon juice

Directions

- Start by heating 1 tablespoon of olive oil on medium-high heat until shimmering without smoke in a large oven.
- Add the celery, carrots, and green onions, toss together.
- Sauté briefly and stir in the garlic.
- Add the chicken broth and bay leaves, immediately increase the heat to high.
- After the liquid is at a rolling boil, add the rice together with the salt and pepper.
- Lower the heat to medium-low let simmer for 20 minutes.
- Stir in the cooked chicken.
- In another separate medium mixing dish, whisk the lemon juice with the eggs.
- Add 2 ladles-full of the broth as you whisk.
- Add the sauce to the chicken soup when it is fully combined, make sure to stir.
- Immediately, remove from heat source.
- Use the fresh parsley for garnishing, if you desire.

Serve and enjoy with bread.

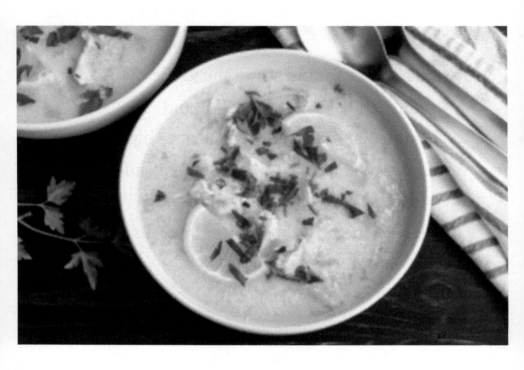

Chunky vegan lentil soup

This recipe entails variety of vegetables and warm spices along with fresh herbs. It is a wonderful one pot Mediterranean Sea diet salad.

Ingredients

- Extra virgin olive oil
- 2 celery stalks, chopped
- 1 cup of chopped fresh parsley, stems removed
- ½ teaspoon of ground cinnamon
- 1 russet potato, small diced
- 1 ½ cups of green lentils
- 4 garlic cloves, chopped
- 1 zucchini squash, diced
- 2 tablespoons of fresh lime or lemon juice
- 1 medium yellow onion, chopped
- Salt and pepper
- 1 teaspoon of ground coriander
- Bread to serve
- 1 bulk carrot, chopped
- 1 teaspoon of ground cumin
- 1 teaspoon of turmeric powder

- ½ teaspoon of cayenne pepper
- 3 cups of canned diced tomatoes with juice
- 2 ½ cup of water
- lime or lemon wedges to serve

Directions

- Place the lentils in a bowl and cover with water.
- Wash and soak for 10 minutes. Drain well.
- In a large heavy pot, heat 2 tablespoons of extra virgin olive oil.
- Add onions, carrot, celery, and potatoes let cook over medium-high heat for 5 minutes, stirring regularly.
- Add garlic and zucchini. Cook for another 5 minutes, stirring regularly.
- Add lentils, salt and pepper and spices.
- Toss to combine, then add the tomatoes and water.
- Bring everything to a boil for 5 minutes.
- Lower the heat cover and let simmer for 20 minutes.

- Remove from heat and stir in parsley and lime juice.
- Transfer to serving bowls and top with a drizzle of <u>extra virgin olive oil</u> .
- Serve and enjoy hot with crusty bread.

Strawberry marshmallow brownies

These Mediterranean Sea diet strawberry marshmallow brownies are chewy on the inside. They are delicious and can make a whole breakfast or as a desert.

Ingredients

- 4 Medium Eggs
- 7 ounces of Marshmallows
- 2 cups of Fresh Strawberries
- 7 ounces of Bittersweet
- 3/4 cup of <u>Granulated Sugar</u>
- 2 teaspoon of Baking Powder
- 11/4 cup of <u>All-Purpose Flour</u>
- 1½ stick of <u>Unsalted Butter</u>

Directions

- Melt the chocolate with butter in a pot containing simmering water.
- Allow it to cool when melted.
- Meanwhile, in a large bowl, whisk eggs, then add sugar. Continue to whisk until foamy.
- Adding in flour with the baking powder.
- Mix until smooth.

- Now, add melted chocolate mix to combined.
- Pour this mixture into a large baking pan that is well aligned with baking paper parchment.
- Then, bake for 10 minutes in a preheated oven at 360°F.
- Top with marshmallows together with the strawberries when the 10 minutes have run out.
- Then move it back in the oven in the same pan.
- Continue to bake another 10 minutes.
- Serve and enjoy when ready.

Fried battered apple rings

This is a simple recipe to make in 5 minutes yet delicious and mouth-watering. Here, apple slices are simply dipped into batter, later deep fried and coated with some cinnamon sugar. It is a wonderful Mediterranean recipe to try at home.

Ingredients

- 11/4 cup of vegetable oil
- ½ cup of all-purpose flour
- 3 tablespoons of milk
- 1 teaspoon of ground cinnamon
- 1/4 cup of granulated sugar
- 1 teaspoon of rum
- 2 large apples
- 1 large egg
- 1 tablespoon of granulated sugar

Directions

- Firstly, combine and mix flour together with the milk, rum, egg, sugar until smooth batter in a soup dish.

- Clean and slice apples into thin slices with the core removed.
- Next, heat up oil in a frying pan until shimmering without smoke.
- Get every ring and dip in the batter and fry until all sides turn to golden brown.
- Fry all the 12 apple slices the same way in 5 minutes or so.
- Drain any excess oil with a kitchen towel.
- Coat in cinnamon sugar before they have cooled completely.
- Serve and enjoy.

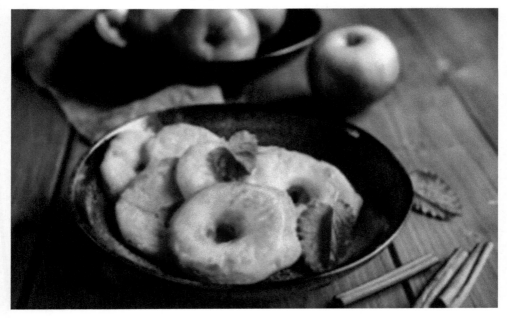

No fuss mixed fruit crisp with hazelnuts

Mediterranean Sea diet emphasizes consumption of vegetable and fruits. Among other several recipes, this no fuss mixed fruit crisp with hazelnuts blends variety of fruits as a tasty desert with fully packed with vitamins.

Ingredients

- 60g of unsalted butter, diced
- 1 kg of mixed fruit mainly apples, peaches, figs
- 20g of unsalted butter
- 100g of plain flour
- 30g of brown sugar
- 2 tablespoons of corn flour
- 50g of hazelnuts , roughly chopped
- 100g of rolled oats
- 40g of brown sugar
- 1 teaspoon of cinnamon

Directions

- Clean the fruits.
- Place all of them into an oven-proof dish.
- Add cinnamon along with hazelnuts, corn flour, and sugar.

- Make sure it is well mixed to spread the ingredients evenly.
- Then, cut the butter into small pieces, place them on top.
- Combine the rolled oats, plain flour, unsalted butter, and brown sugar in a larger bowl.
- Mix thoroughly to combine with your hands.
- Incorporate the butter into the oats mixture.
- Break up the butter blend into the into oats.
- Spread the topping evenly over the fruits.
- Put in a preheated oven to bake for 45 minutes over high heat until the juices just begin to bubble.
- Serve and enjoy with ice cream.

Strawberry banana frozen yogurt

The Mediterranean Sea diet has invented many substitutions to consumption of unhealthy foods. This strawberry banana frozen yogurt is a perfect replacement for ice cream that has high sugar and calorie content.

Ingredients

- 2 tablespoon of honey
- 2 ripe bananas
- Frozen strawberries
- Greek yogurt

Directions

- Firstly, place the strawberries to thaw a bit.
- Then puree in a food processor.
- Place in the peeled and sliced bananas to the mixture.
- Add the yogurt to the mixture continue to process until smooth.
- Taste and adjust accordingly.
- Transfer into a plastic container when tightly covered with a lid.
- Place in freezer and let freeze.

- Remove the container after 2 hours.
- Break the ice with a spoon.
- Serve and enjoy with your required consistency.

No bake banana banoffee pie

This Mediterranean Sea diet is quite flourless and with no eggs as well. the desert only blends bananas as the main flavor to this desert.

Ingredients

- Chocolate
- 1 can of Dulce de Leche
- 10 ounces of Whipping Cream
- 2 Bananas
- ½ cup of Melted butter
- 2 tablespoons Icing Sugar
- 8.8 ounces of Digestive Biscuits

Directions

- Expressly, begin by melting the butter.
- Crush the biscuits into crumbs in a food processor.
- Then, pour over the melted butter let mix until well combined.
- Line the bottom and sides of a round cake tin with baking paper.

- Place two thirds of the biscuit mix in. Make sure to spread the mix evenly.
- Out of the paper, cut a circle and place it over the biscuit crumbs.
- Press down hard enough with your hands to create an even base.
- After this, feel free to discard the baking paper.
- Add biscuit crumbs on the sides of the cake tin, but ensure to create a wall with a spoon.
- Transfer the mixture to refrigerate for 30 minutes.
- As the mixture refrigerates, pour half of the Dulce de Leech into a sauce pan.
- Bring to a boil for 5 minutes, stirring constantly.
- Let it cool little bit.
- Spread it over the chilled biscuit base.
- The remaining half of Dulce de Leche should now be used to spread over the thick layer.
- Cover with the banana slices.
- Pour chilled cream into a chilled dish.
- Now, add icing sugar and whip to make it stiff.

- Spread the cream over the banana layer.
- Place back in the fridge for 1 hour.
- If desired, finish with chocolate shavings.
- Serve and enjoy.

Plum tart with ricotta and Greek yogurt

Ingredients

- 100g of ricotta
- 2 teaspoons of ground cinnamon
- 60g of unsalted butter
- 100g of Greek yogurt
- 2 tablespoons of powdered sugar
- 100g of superfine sugar
- 2 medium eggs
- 2 teaspoons of baking powder
- 160g of all-purpose flour
- 400g of plums

Directions

- Begin by creaming your butter with sugar for about 5 minutes or so.
- Add eggs, one at a time and beat preferably with an electric mixer until fluffy.
- Place in the ricotta into Greek yogurt and mix.
- Then, sift in the flour mixed together with the baking powder and cinnamon.

- Fold in with a wooden spoon to combine all ingredients.
- Cut the plumbs in half after cleaning and remove pits.
- Place onto a baking tray and pour the mixture in the pan, for a silicone cake pan.
- Spread the mixture evenly them top with the plums.
- Proceed to bake for 40 minutes in a preheated oven at 350°F.
- Remove from the oven when ready and let cool totally.
- Dust with some icing sugar.
- Serve and enjoy.

Tahini banana shakes

This banana shakes recipe takes about 5 minutes to make. Interestingly, it can be made ahead of time, but trust me, you will not rest until you have consumed it all at once because of sweetness and irresistible taste.

Ingredients

- 2 sliced frozen bananas
- 4 pitted Medjool dates
- 1/4 cup tahini
- 1/4 cup crushed ice
- 1 ½ cups unsweetened almond milk
- Pinch ground cinnamon

Directions

- Begin by adding the sliced frozen bananas in a blender along with the remaining ingredients at once.
- Keep the blender until a visible smooth and creamy shake.
- Transfer the date shakes to your serving cups.
- Add the pinch ground cinnamon on the top of the cream.

- Enjoy

How to freezing the bananas?

- Slice peeled bananas in to 2 slices.
- Arrange the banana slices in one layer put on a lined sheet pan with parchment paper
- Put in the freezer until the bananas are completely frozen.
- Transfer the frozen bananas to a freezer safe bag and or close tightly in case you want to use at a later time.

The ultimate Mediterranean breakfast

If one is looking for a wholesomely satisfying breakfast, then look not for the answer, it is right here. This breakfast can be packed with falafel, baba ganoush, hummus, and tabbouleh.

Ingredients

- 1 Baba Ganoush Recipe
- Grapes
- Feta cheese
- Extra virgin olive oil and Za'atar to dip
- Pita Bread, sliced into quarters
- 1 Tabbouleh Recipe
- Marinated artichokes or mushrooms
- 1 to 2 tomatoes, sliced
- 1 English cucumber, sliced
- 6 to 7 sliced Radish
- 1 Falafel Recipe
- Assorted olives
- Fresh herbs for garnish
- 1 Classic Hummus Recipe

Directions

- Begin by preparing the falafel recipe at least a night before mainly soaking the chickpeas. Alternatively, one can simply buy the ready falafel.

- Also make the hummus recipe and baba ganoush, a night prior and store in a refrigerator.

- Slice the feta cheese a head of time.

- Make the tabouli in advance. It is okay if it is made days prior but must be kept in tight-lid container and refrigerated.

- To assemble, put the baba ganoush, olive oil, za'atar, hummus, and the tabouli in bowls.

- The largest bowl should be place at the center of a platter for the purposes of creating an easy focal point.

- Place other bowls besides the largest bowl to form shape and easy movement.

- Using the gaps between the bowls, place the remaining ingredients; sliced vegetables, falafel, and pita bread.

- Add the grapes and do not forget to garnish with herbs if desired.
- Serve and enjoy.

Frozen banana pops

Ingredients

- 2 teaspoons chia seeds
- 4 teaspoons freeze dried raspberries
- 4 bananas
- 2 teaspoons pollen
- 2 tablespoons almond butter
- 1 cup Greek yogurt
- 1/4 cup almonds without skin and roughly chopped

Directions

- Cut bananas into halves and place on a tray lined with baking parchment let them freeze for 30 minutes.
- As it freezes, combine the Greek yogurt together with the almond butter and blend well.
- Stick the bananas with an ice pop after you have removed them from the fridge.
- Coat each with yogurt mixture, then place it onto the tray.

- Do this for all the bananas.
- Sprinkle with freeze dried raspberries, chopped almonds, pollen and chia seeds.
- Return the tray back to the freezer to let set for an hour.
- Serve and enjoy when frozen.

Vegan peanut butter banana brownies

If you have never tested a flourless banana brownie, this is your chance to make one for your own. It is gluten free and rich in protein content. Is features dates and banana which are kept fudgy

Ingredients

- 2 cups of pitted dates
- 1/4 cup of coconut oil , melted
- 2 tablespoon of water
- ⅓ cup of unsweetened cocoa powder
- ⅓ cup of peanut butter
- 1 large banana, ripe
- A pinch of salt

Directions

- Preheat your oven to 356°F
- Place the dates, coconut oil, and water in a food processor.
- Process until it forms a paste.
- Add cocoa powder, banana, peanut butter, and salt after it has formed the paste.
- Process until smooth.

- Shift the entire mixture into a pan lined with baking parchment.
- Then, bake for 10 minutes.
- Let cool when ready.
- Slice and enjoy.

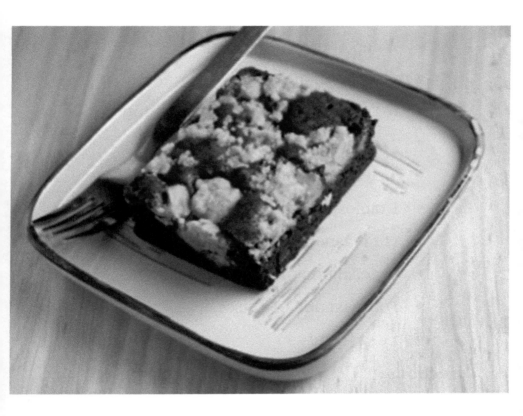

Spiced cocoa roasted almonds

This is mainly a snack recipe. They are very delicious especially when covered with cocoa.

Ingredients

- 2 tablespoons of brown sugar
- 1 tablespoon of water
- ½ cup of brown sugar
- 1 teaspoon of ground cinnamon
- 1/4 teaspoon of ground cinnamon
- 7 ounces of almonds , raw
- ½ teaspoon of ground nutmeg
- 1 tablespoon of unsweetened cocoa powder
- 1/4 teaspoon of cardamom
- ½ teaspoon of sea salt
- 1/4 teaspoon of anise
- 1 egg white

Directions

- Combine the egg white with water and whisk until frothy.
- Add sugar together with the spices and salt mix thoroughly.

- Place in the almonds blend well to coat.
- Transfer the mixture to a baking tray aligned with baking parchment.
- Spread the mixture around in one layer.
- Bake in a preheated oven at 300°F for 30 minutes.
- Endeavor to stir as it bakes gently.
- Shift the roasted almonds into a sauce pan with cocoa, sugar, cinnamon.
- Shake the mixture with the lid closed to coat the almond.
- Let cool.
- Serving and enjoy.

Double chocolate oatmeal

Chocolate oatmeal is a recipe with rich carbohydrate content and fiber making it a perfect Mediterranean Sea diet choice for an energy giving breakfast. It is chocolate flavored sweetened with honey or syrup topping with strawberries.

Ingredients

- 1/4 cup of chocolate chips
- 12 fresh strawberries
- 1 cup of water
- A pinch of salt
- 1 cup of milk
- 4 tablespoons of maple syrup
- 1 cup of rolled oats
- 2 tablespoon of unsweetened cocoa powder

Directions

- Roll the oats, together milk, salt and water in a pot.
- Bring to a boil when covered.
- Lower the heat and open the lid.

- Add cocoa powder and stir frequently for 7minutes.
- Stir in the maple syrup and chocolate chips when the heat is turned off.
- Place in 2 serving dishes.
- Serve when topped with strawberries and chocolate chips.
- Enjoy.

Quinoa egg muffins

Eggs are known for the provision of most food nutrients. They are juicy and very flavorful for a delicious breakfast.

Ingredients

- a pinch of black pepper
- 1 large carrot, grated
- ½ tsp salt
- ½ leek, chopped
- 1 green pepper, diced
- 3 ounce of cheddar cheese, grated
- 2 tablespoons of Greek yogurt
- ½ zucchini
- 2 tablespoons of dried oregano
- 2 tablespoons of extra virgin olive oil
- ½ cup of uncooked quinoa
- 2 eggs, small-medium

Directions

- Preheat your oven at 350°F.
- Start by cooking quinoa as per the manufacturers package Directions.
- Let cool briefly.

- Heat olive oil in the frying pan.
- Add chopped leek, diced pepper, grated carrot, and diced zucchini let Sauté for 10 minutes.
- Stir in the oregano.
- Season with salt accordingly.
- In a bowl, beat the eggs mixing with the yogurt, and salt.
- Add black pepper, grated cheese, and cooled quinoa.
- Add sautéed veggies mix thoroughly to blend and combine.
- Align a muffin tray with paper
- Place the mixture in all the spots in the tray.
- Bake in the preheated oven for 20 minutes.
- Serve and enjoy.

Sweet potato burgers

Sweet potato burger is a whole meal Mediterranean Sea diet vegetable burger made with buckwheat.

Ingredients

- Guacamole
- ½ cup of buckwheat
- 1 tablespoon of <u>curry powder</u>
- 2 large tomatoes
- 1 small onion
- 2 carrots
- ½ cucumber
- 3 cups of diced sweet potatoes
- 2 tablespoons of <u>extra virgin olive oil</u>
- 1/4 red cabbage
- Salt and pepper to taste
- ½ cup of packed fresh parsley
- 6 buns

Directions

- Place the sweet potatoes in a sauce pan.
- Add in water to cover them all.
- Boil covered with lid.

- After it has boiled for 6 minutes, lower the heat and continue to cook until soft in 4 minutes or so.
- Drain any excess water and set aside.
- As the potatoes are cooking, cook the buckwheat following the package Directions.
- Sauté onions and carrots in a skillet with some olive oil until onions are translucent.
- Shift the potatoes into a mixing bowl.
- Using a potato masher, mash them with a fork.
- Introduce the remaining ingredients and mix well.
- Use part of the mixture and roll it into a ball.
- Move it onto a baking tray.
- Make sure the tray is aligned with parchment paper.
- Repeat this for all the mixture.
- Bake in already heated oven at 360°F for 10 minutes.
- Turn the other side, continue to bake for another 10 minutes.
- Serve with buns and lots of veggies.

Blueberry coffee breakfast smoothie

The exciting flavor of coffee takes control of this smoothie. It features blueberry with natural sweetness for a healthy and tasty breakfast.

Ingredients

- 6 <u>dates</u> , pitted
- ½ cup of <u>rolled oats</u>
- 2 teaspoons of <u>instant coffee</u>
- 1 cup of almond milk
- 1 cup of fresh blueberries

Directions

- In a blender, combine the oats together with the blueberries, dates, instant coffee, and milk.
- Bland until finely smooth.
- Serve and enjoy immediately.

Apricot coconut popsicles

Apricot coconut popsicles are frozen treat with a refreshing healthy taste and so easy and quick to make in 10 minutes.

Ingredients

- 3 tablespoons of coconut oil
- 3 tablespoons of honey
- 1/4 cup of coconut milk
- 2 cups of apricots, pitted and halved

Directions

- Place all ingredients in a food processor, process until smooth.
- Pour the mixture into the popsicle molds with inserted sticks.
- Freeze for not less than 4 hours.
- Serve and enjoy.

793. Cherry avocado chocolate mousse

This is a perfect healthy desert with no added artificial sugar. These cherry avocado chocolate mousse features a rich chocolate flavor, creamy avocado and cherries and dates from where it derives its sweetness.

Ingredients

- ⅛ teaspoon of pink salt
- ½ cup of coconut milk drink
- 1 cup of cherries, stoned
- ½ cup of dates
- 2 large avocados
- ½ cup of natural unsweetened cocoa powder

Directions

- Start by soaking the dates in water for 30 minutes.
- Cut avocados in half.
- Using a spoon, scoop out the flesh, put in a food processor.
- Add cocoa powder together with the dates, coconut milk drink, cherries, and salt.
- Process until smooth and creamy.
- Use the cherries to beautify.
- Serve and enjoy.

Ricotta chocolate banana toast with seeds

This breakfast can keep you until your next meal time. It is basically a whole wheat toast in 10 minutes.

Ingredients

- 2 teaspoons of honey
- 1 cup ricotta
- 4 slices of toast bread
- 4 teaspoons of mixed seed
- 2 large bananas
- 2 ounces of dark chocolate

Directions

- Begin by toasting your bread using a toaster.
- Combine ricotta with honey as the bread toasts.
- Taste and adjust accordingly.
- Melt the chocolate over a pot of simmering water.
- Spread it over every toasted bread.
- Add ricotta mixture with the sliced banana and seeds.
- If you like, garnish with grated chocolate.

- Serve and enjoy.

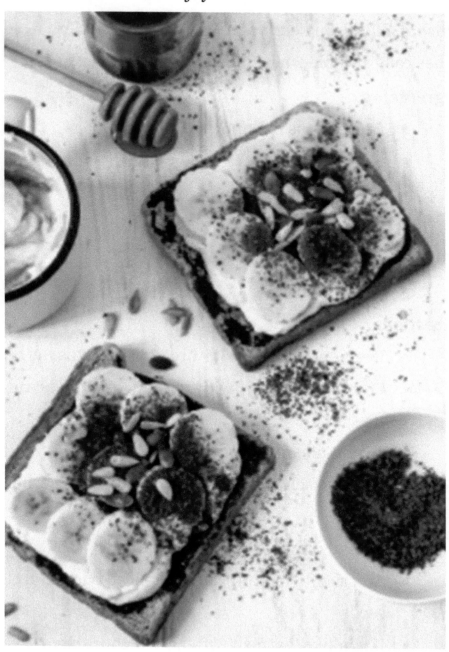

Homemade strawberry jam with brown sugar

The uniqueness with this recipe is that it has no artificial preservatives making it a health Mediterranean diet for a breakfast.

Ingredients

- 2.2 pounds of strawberries
- 1½ lemon
- ½ pound of brown sugar

Directions

- Hull the strawberries and cut into small pieces.
- Refrigerate in a bowl.
- Place in a large pot. Stir with vigor for 5 minutes over medium heat.
- Make sure they turn mushy.
- Add sugar together with the lemon juice.
- Cook for 35 minutes or until the jam is thick while stirring frequently.
- It is time to remove the saucer from the fridge.
- Spread with some jam.

- Let it cool down and check its thickness by drawing a line through.
- Cook it further, if the jam does not fill the space of the drawn line.
- Otherwise, pour into sterilized jugs leaving 1 cm free from the top.
- Seal properly, then turn up-side down.
- Let it settle for at least 30 minutes.
- Return the jugs to an upright position.
- Serve and enjoy.

Blueberry turnovers

The recipe combines puff pastry together with homemade blueberry fillings. This Mediterranean diet is fit for breakfast, lunch or dinner.

Ingredients

- All-purpose flour , for dusting
- ⅓ cup brown sugar
- 1 tablespoon lemon juice
- 1 teaspoon brown sugar
- 1 small egg, beaten
- 2 ounces unsalted butter
- 2 teaspoons cornstarch
- 1 sheet puff pastry, thawed or fresh
- 2 cups frozen blueberries

Directions

- Combine blueberries, sugar with the lemon juice and simmer for 10 minutes in a small saucepan.
- Follow by stirring in the butter.
- Make sure to dilute cornstarch in 1 tablespoon of water in a cup.

- Add bit of the blueberry sauce, stir well to mix.
- Pour the cornstarch into the saucepan, make sure to stir until the sauce is thick.
- Pour it into a bowl when ready, let cool for 30 minutes.
- Preheat an oven to 400°F.
- Unfold the puff pastry and roll it out.
- Cut into squares.
- Scoop 2 heaped teaspoons blueberry filling in the middle of pastry squares.
- Run your finger alongside the sides of each square after dipping your finger in water.
- Lift one tip of the pastry and fold it over the filling towards the opposite tip forming a triangle.
- To seal, press down the edges.
- Double-seal with a fork.
- Place turnovers onto a baking tray.
- Pierce each turnover to allow steam to escape.
- Brush with egg wash and sprinkle with brown sugar.
- Bake in the oven for 15 minutes and serve.

Strawberry coconut tart

This recipe uses simple and easy to find ingredients. It is quite easy to make from scratch in 35 minutes.

Ingredients

- 2/3 cups of unsweetened desiccated coconut
- 1 stick unsalted butter , melted
- 4 tablespoons of strawberry jam
- 3 tablespoons of powdered sugar
- 1 cup of all-purpose flour
- ½ cup of powdered sugar
- 1 egg white, from a large egg

Directions

- In a mixing bowl, combine flour with powdered sugar.
- Add melted butter.
- Make sure to mix thoroughly with a large spoon.
- Mix your hands when it begins to form dough.
- Wrap it and let chill for 30 minutes.
- Remove it from the fridge and fill the bottom and sides of a pie pan with it. Do not roll.

- Take a piece of the pastry and press it down. This should be piece by piece until you use up all of it.
- Spread jam over the crust. Keep aside.
- Whip the egg white until soft peaks appear.
- Add sifted sugar and beat until smooth.
- Stir in the coconut.
- Pour this mixture over the jam and spread evenly round.
- Bake in a preheated oven at 350°F for 25-30 minutes.
- Remove out when ready and let it cool totally.
- Serve and enjoy.

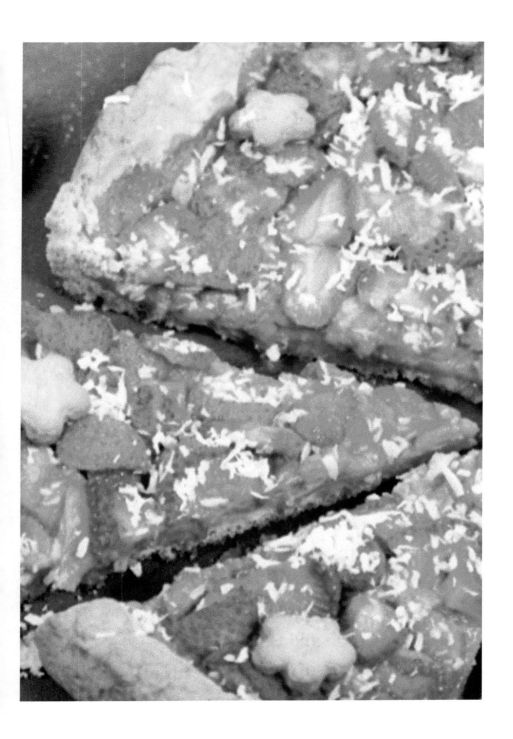

Mango panna cotta

Though a perfect Mediterranean Sea diet, mango panna cotta an Italian desert wonderful picnics, parties and dinners. It can be prepared ahead of time.

Ingredients

- A knob of butter
- ½ cup of whole milk
- ½ teaspoon of vanilla essence
- 1 cup of heavy cream the whole package
- 1 packet gelatin
- ½ lemon, juice only
- 2 cups of frozen mango chunks, thawed
- ⅓ cup of granulated sugar
- 2 tablespoons of granulated sugar

Directions

- Pour heavy cream together with the milk and sugar into a small sauce pan.
- Stir to dissolve the sugar on over low heat, the cream should be hot.
- Turn off the heat and stir vanilla essence. Make sure not to boil at this stage.

- The bloom should be gelatin as per the package Directions.
- Add the bloomed gelatin to the cooled cream mixture. Do not forget to mix to dissolve.
- Pour the mixture into small glasses, place to refrigerate to set the panna cotta for 2 hours.
- Process the thawed mango pieces together with the lemon juice and sugar in a blender until smooth.
- Taste and adjust accordingly.
- Simmer in a small saucepan over low heat.
- Stir in butter to get a much creamier texture.
- Allow the mixture to cool.
- Pour over the panna cotta.
- Serve and enjoy.

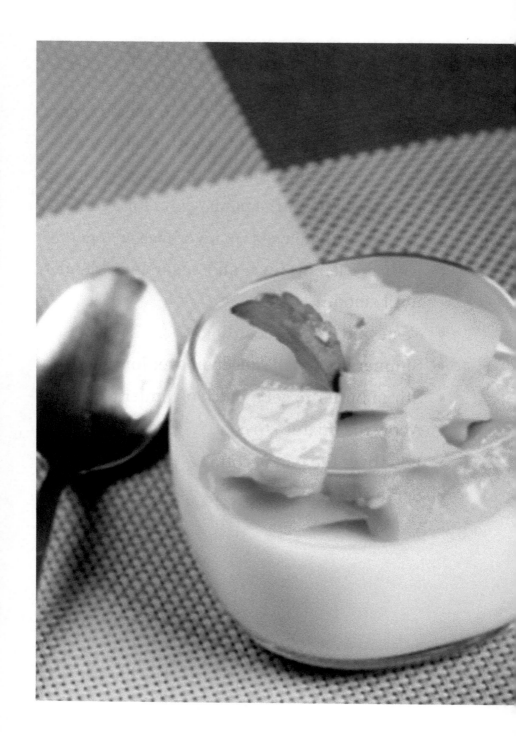

Candied oranges dipped in chocolate

This recipe is for a sweet tasty treat for a perfect holiday to enjoy Mediterranean Sea diet. The chocolates can be substituted with cupcakes if you like.

Ingredients

- 3.5 ounces of Dark Chocolate
- 1 Large Orange, organic
- Coarse Salt
- 1 cup of Granulated Sugar
- 1 cup of Water

Directions

- Cut the oranges into thin slices.
- Heat water and sugar in a large pot until the sugar has dissolved.
- Add the orange slices in a manner that they are spread around without covering each other totally.
- Let simmer for 40 minutes on a low heat. Turn occasionally.
- Transfer slices onto a wire rack when ready, let them cool completely.

- It is fine to cool on a fridge to speed up the cooling process.
- Melt the chocolate over a pot of simmering water.
- Dip half of each slice in chocolate.
- Place the dipped one's onto a tray lined with a sheet of aluminum foil.
- Sprinkle with salt.
- Shift all of them into the fridge.
- Serve an enjoy.

Walnut crescent cookies

If you want taste and know divine taste covered in a powdered sugar, look no further, walnut crescent cookies can give you that same exact taste.

Ingredients

- 2 tablespoons of vanilla sugar
- 11/4 cup of all-purpose flour
- ½ cup of powdered sugar
- 1 stick unsalted butter
- ⅔ cup of ground walnuts
- 4 tablespoons of powdered sugar
- 1 teaspoon of vanilla essence

Directions

- In a large mixing bowl, begin by combining sifted powdered sugar, sifted flour, and ground walnuts.
- Next, add vanilla essence and mix thoroughly.
- Then, grate chilled butter.
- Add to the bowl.

- Combine all the ingredients using your bare hands until dough is formed in 3 minutes or so.
- Place into a Ziploc bag allow it to chill for 30 minutes in the fridge.
- As it refrigerates, get a small bowl and place extra powdered sugar with vanilla sugar in it and keep aside.
- Take a piece of the dough and roll into a ball then into a sausage.
- Shape the sausage into a crescent.
- Place onto a baking tray with baking parchment.
- For the remaining dough, repeat this step.
- Bake in a ready heated oven at 400°F for 8 minutes or so.
- Allow it to cool down completely on the tray when already fried.
- Transfer to a plat and dip with powdered sugar to coat.
- Serve and enjoy.

Banana bread

Banana is a fruit of the heart blessed with abundant fiber. Above and beyond, it is moist, soft and sweet. It is best with honey or butter depending on how you like it.

Ingredients

- A few drops of vanilla essence
- ½ cup of granulated sugar
- 1 large egg
- 1½ cup of all-purpose flour
- 1 teaspoon of baking soda
- 3 large ripe bananas
- ⅓ cup of unsalted butter
- 1 teaspoon of ground cinnamon

Directions

- Begin by preparing the bananas, cut them into small pieces.
- Put them in a medium sized dish, then mash them with a fork.
- Add in large egg, beaten with a fork. Mix properly.

- Add baking soda along with the melted butter, caster sugar, vanilla essence, flour. Make sure you mix well.
- Pour the batter into a loaf tin lined with baking paper.
- Place in a preheated oven and bake for 1 hour at 355°F.
- Serve and enjoy.

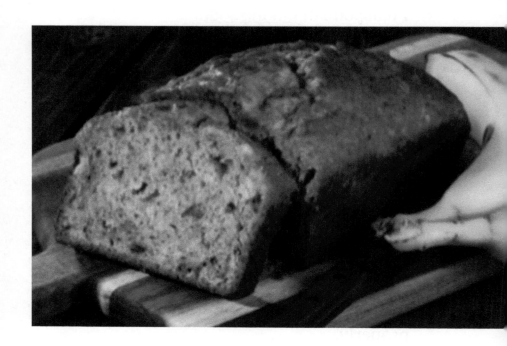

Apple oatmeal bake

Oat is a nutritious ingredient, on the other hand, apple is a healthy fruit that can help to keep the doctor away. As a result, this recipe is a healthy Mediterranean Sea diet rich with fruits and whole foods especially oats.

Ingredients

- ⅔ cup of granulated sugar
- 2 cups of rolled oats
- 2 teaspoons of cinnamon
- 1½ stick of unsalted butter
- 1 cup of walnuts
- 6 large apples

Directions

- In a food processor, process the oats and walnuts until you get flour-like texture.
- Grate the apples with fruit grater.
- In a mixing dish, mix the processed oats together with, walnuts, and sugar.
- Next, oil your ovenproof dish with butter.
- Use the oat mixture to cover the bottom of the oven dish.

- Press down slightly to add half of the apples.
- Cover with more oat mixture on top.
- Repeat this step until everything is done.
- Slice the butter after which cover the whole surface with it.
- Proceed to bake for 35 minutes in a preheated oven at 400°F until golden brown.
- Serve and pour over vanilla pudding if you like.
- Enjoy.

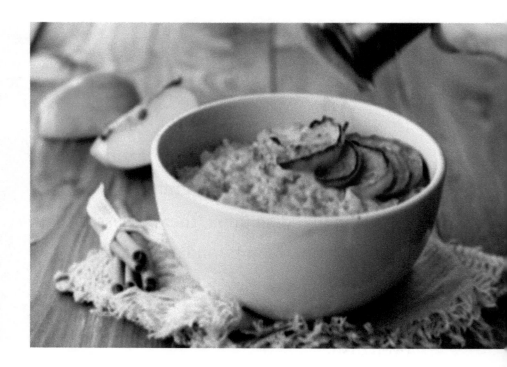

Plum tart with ricotta and Greek yogurt

Ingredients

- 100g of ricotta
- 2 teaspoons of ground cinnamon
- 60g of unsalted butter
- 100g of Greek yogurt
- 2 tablespoons of powdered sugar
- 100g of superfine sugar
- 2 medium eggs
- 2 teaspoons of baking powder
- 160g of all-purpose flour
- 400g of plums

Directions

- Begin by creaming your butter with sugar for about 5 minutes or so.
- Add eggs, one at a time and beat preferably with an electric mixer until fluffy.
- Place in the ricotta into Greek yogurt and mix.
- Then, sift in the flour mixed together with the baking powder and cinnamon.

- Fold in with a wooden spoon to combine all ingredients.
- Cut the plumbs in half after cleaning and remove pits.
- Place onto a baking tray and pour the mixture in the pan, for a silicone cake pan.
- Spread the mixture evenly them top with the plums.
- Proceed to bake for 40 minutes in a preheated oven at 350°F.
- Remove from the oven when ready and let cool totally.
- Dust with some icing sugar.
- Serve and enjoy.

Chocolate Nutella Mousse with strawberries

This is a desert with an exciting tasty and sweetness for any occasion. It is easy and quick to make in only 30 minutes, you will be exciting your taste buds with this Mediterranean Sea diet recipe.

Ingredients

- 2 tablespoons of lemon juice
- 2 cups of whipping cream
- 2 tablespoons of caster sugar
- 7 ounces of dark chocolate
- 2 cups of fresh strawberries
- 2 tablespoons of powdered sugar
- 5 tablespoons of Nutella

Directions

- Start by cutting the chocolate into small pieces.
- Over double boiler melt the chocolates with ½ cup of whipping cream. Allow it to cool.

- As the chocolate melts, whip the cream together with the powdered sugar until soft peaks form.
- Then, whisk Nutella with a few tablespoons of whipped cream in a large mixing dish.
- Fold the whipped cream into the Nutella mixture.
- It is time to stir in the cooled chocolate.
- Divide the mousse into 5 glasses or more.
- Place in the refrigerator for 60 minutes.
- As the mousse refrigerates, prepare the strawberries by cleaning, and trimming any green parts.
- Cut into small pieces.
- Shift them into a bowl.
- Add caster sugar and lemon juice.
- Place in a refrigerator 30 minutes.
- Remove and top each glass with strawberries and the juice if any.
- Serve and enjoy.

No bake pineapple cake with Nutella

This incredible desert recipe only features 7 ingredients and gets ready in 20 minutes; a very short time, isn't it? This recipe can be made ahead of time with Nutella and pineapple pieces.

Ingredients

- 1 can of pineapple slices
- 1 ½ cup of sour cream
- 4 tablespoons of Nutella
- 2 tablespoons of powdered sugar
- ½ cup of Greek yogurt
- ½ cup of sour cream
- 3 tablespoons of powdered sugar
- 2 cups of graham crumbs, heaped
- ⅓ cup of unsalted butter

Directions

- Mix melted butter together with the digestive biscuit crumbs. Endeavor to combine well.
- Shift the entire mixture into cake tin, press down to make the crust.

- Drain the pineapple slices of any excess unwanted water and pat them dry.
- Cut 4 – 5 pineapple slices in halves.
- Place them inside the cake pan with others (they should be separate; they should touch each other).
- Any remaining pineapples should be cut into small pieces and spread them over the biscuit layer.
- Whisk together powdered sugar with Nutella and the Sour cream to combined.
- Spread this mixture over the pineapple slices.
- Now, in another separate mixing dish, mix sour cream together with the powdered sugar, and Greek yogurt.
- Spread over Nutella layer.
- Cover this mixture with cling film.
- Move it to the fridge, let refrigerate for at 14 hours.
- You can beautify with pineapples if you like.
- Serve and enjoy.

Lightning Source UK Ltd.
Milton Keynes UK
UKHW020749030621
384855UK00001B/76